I0791454

Your Free Gift

Sometimes it can get a bit confusing as to what's keto, and should I try it or not? I hope my short book gives you a clear understanding of the Keto's world. And if you liked it and you want to move on, I have great news for you!

Right now, I'm writing a full **Ketogenic Diet For Beginners' guide** and **cookbook**, and if you want to get the books right away, please click on this link and follow the instructions.

Thanks!

Alena Bri

Table of Contents

What can I eat and what is not?

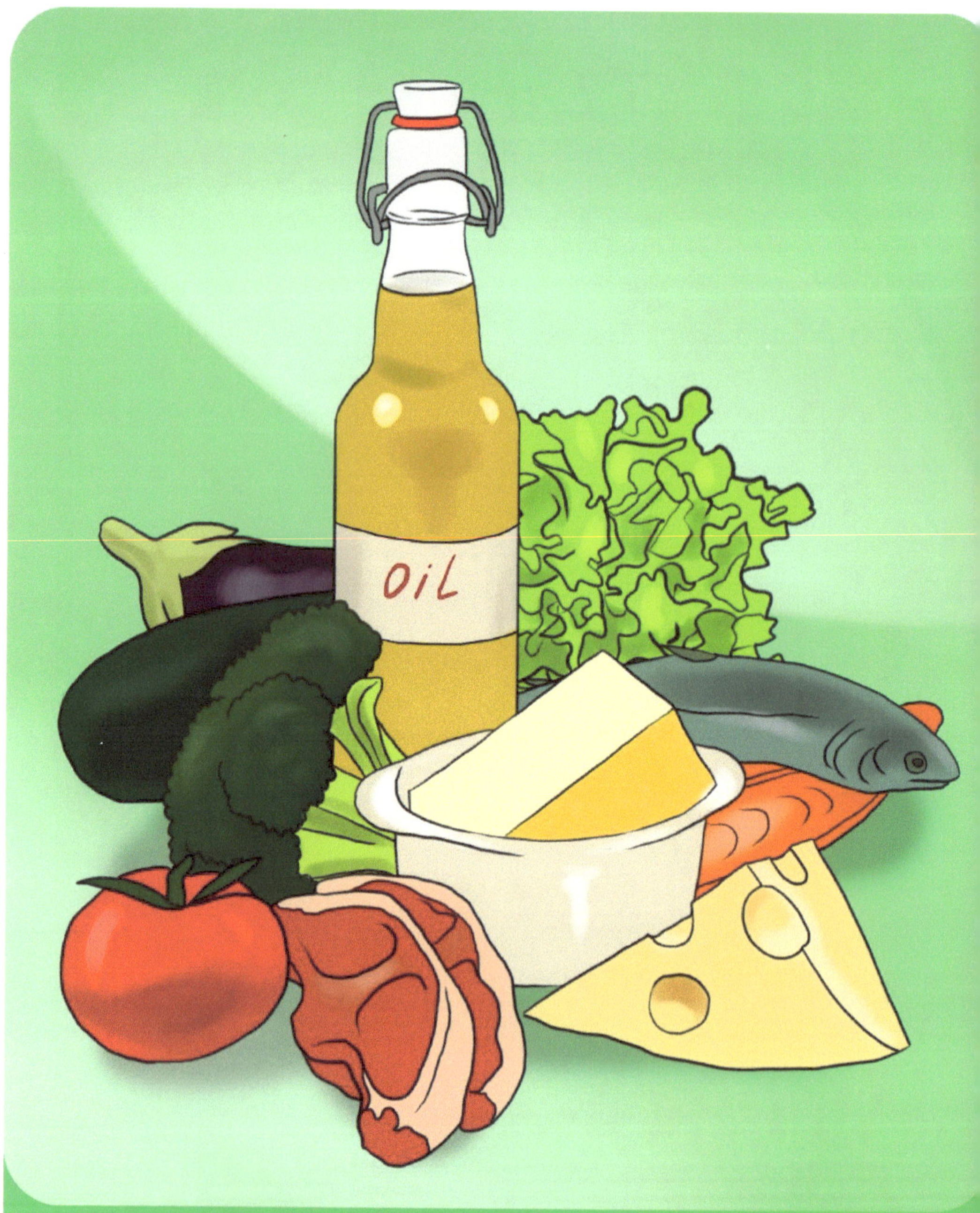

Eat real food

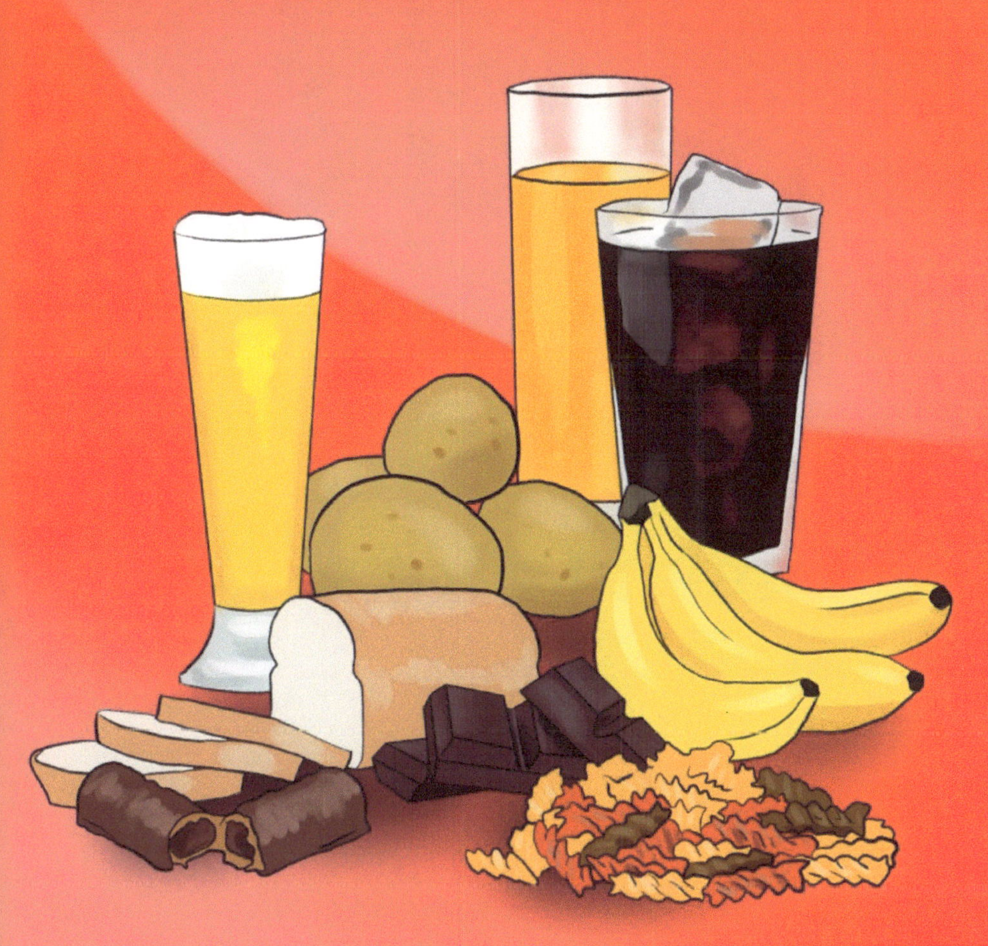

Avoid sugar and starch

Amazing health benefits for you!

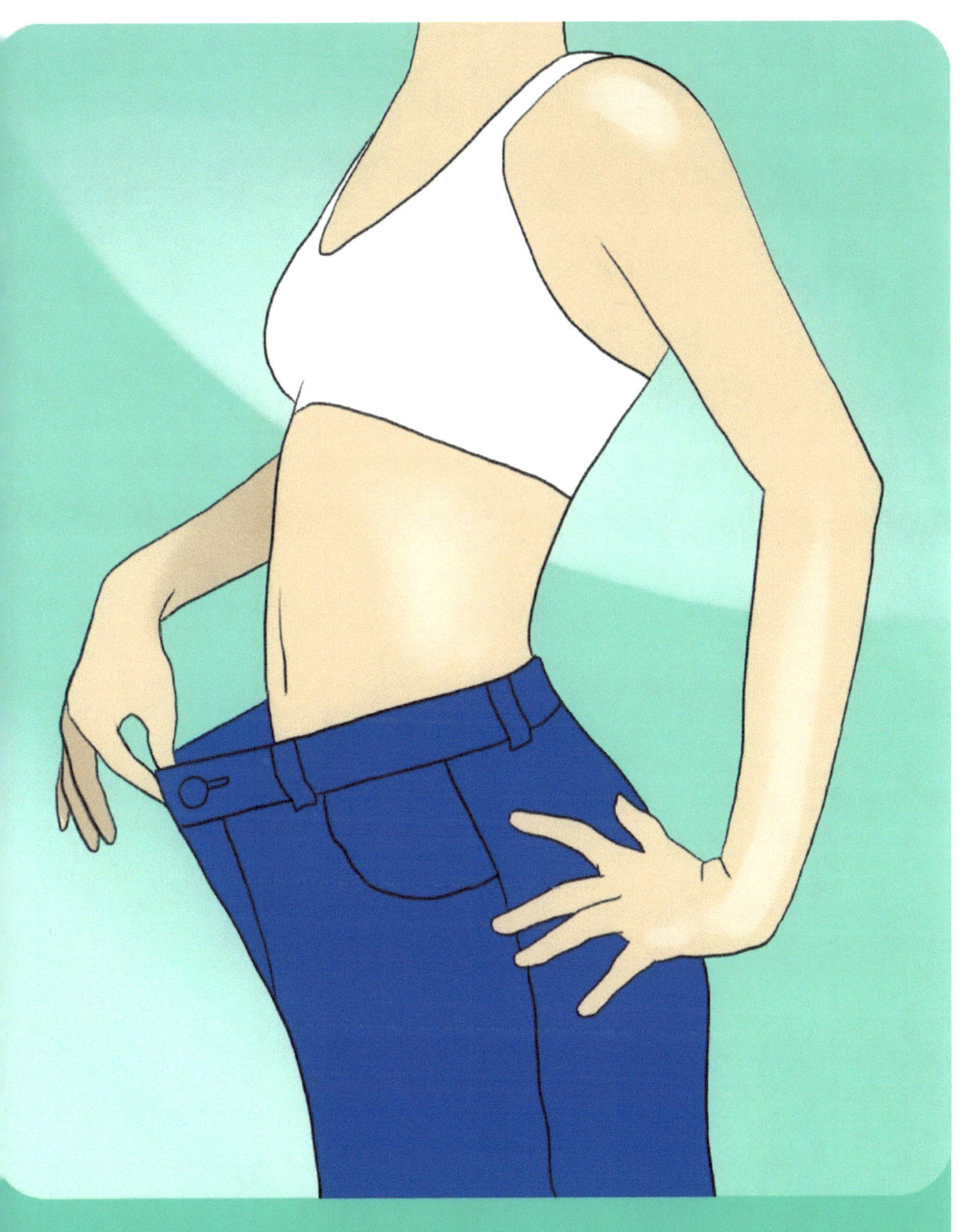

Lose weight

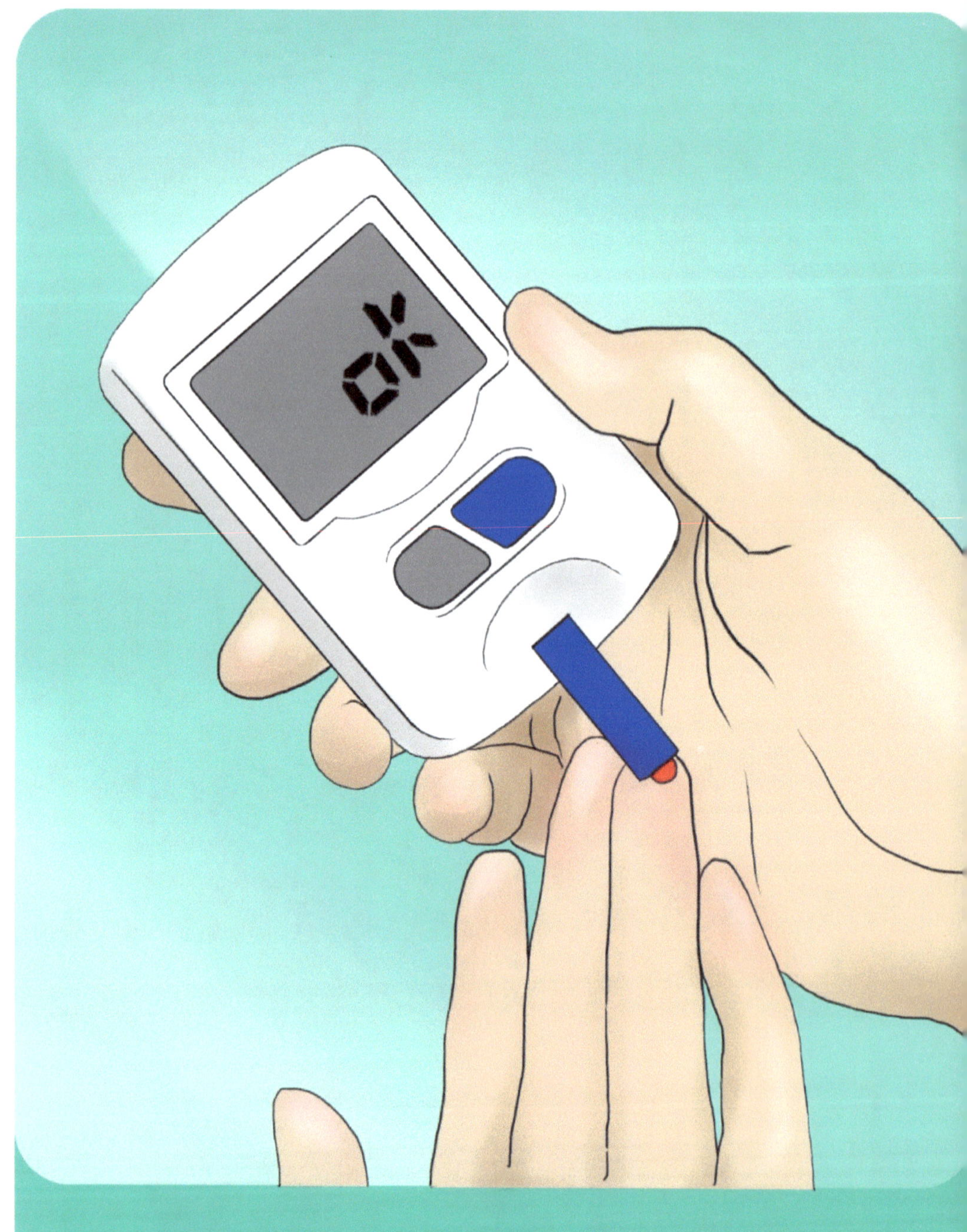

Reverse your type 2 diabetes

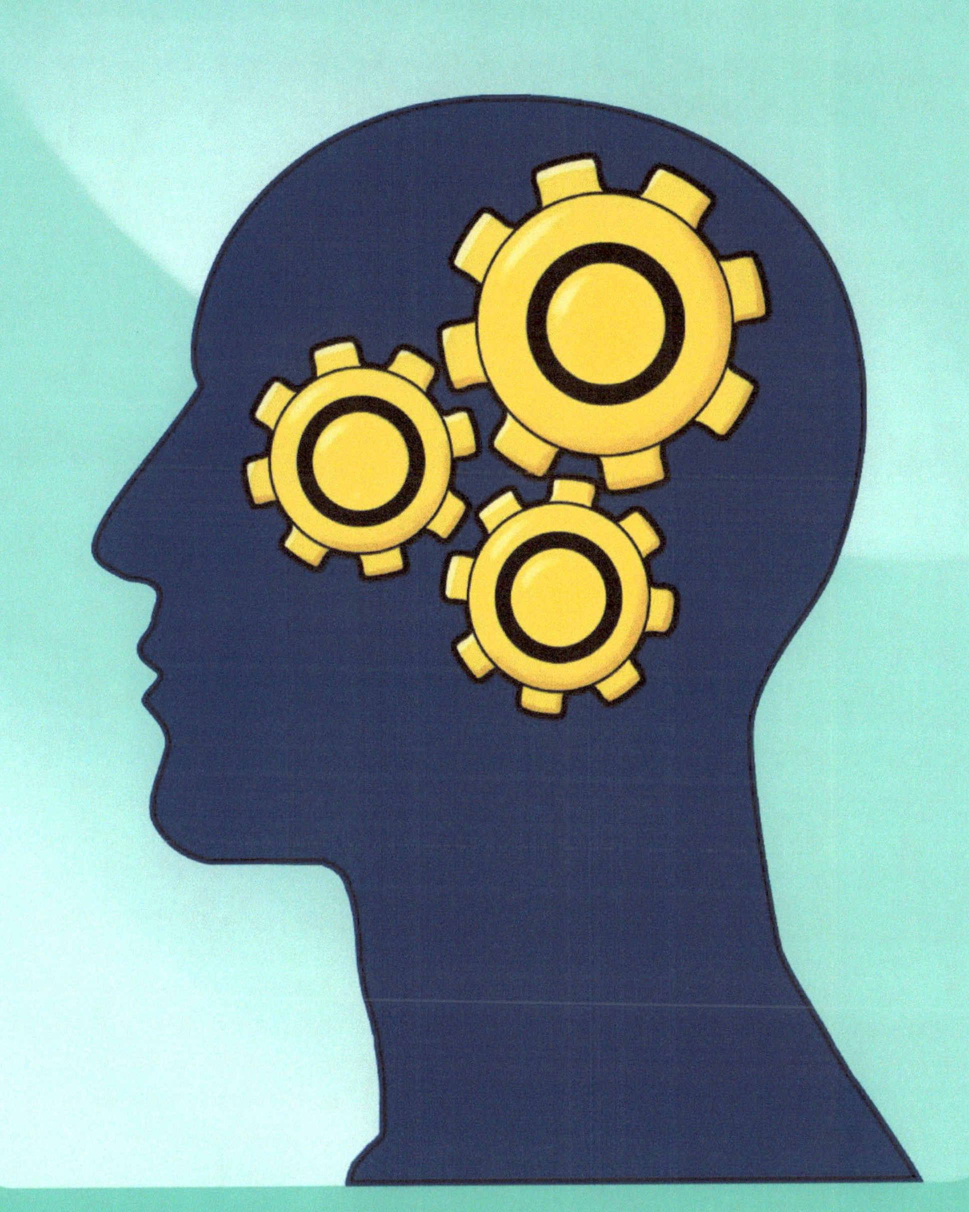

Boost
brain health

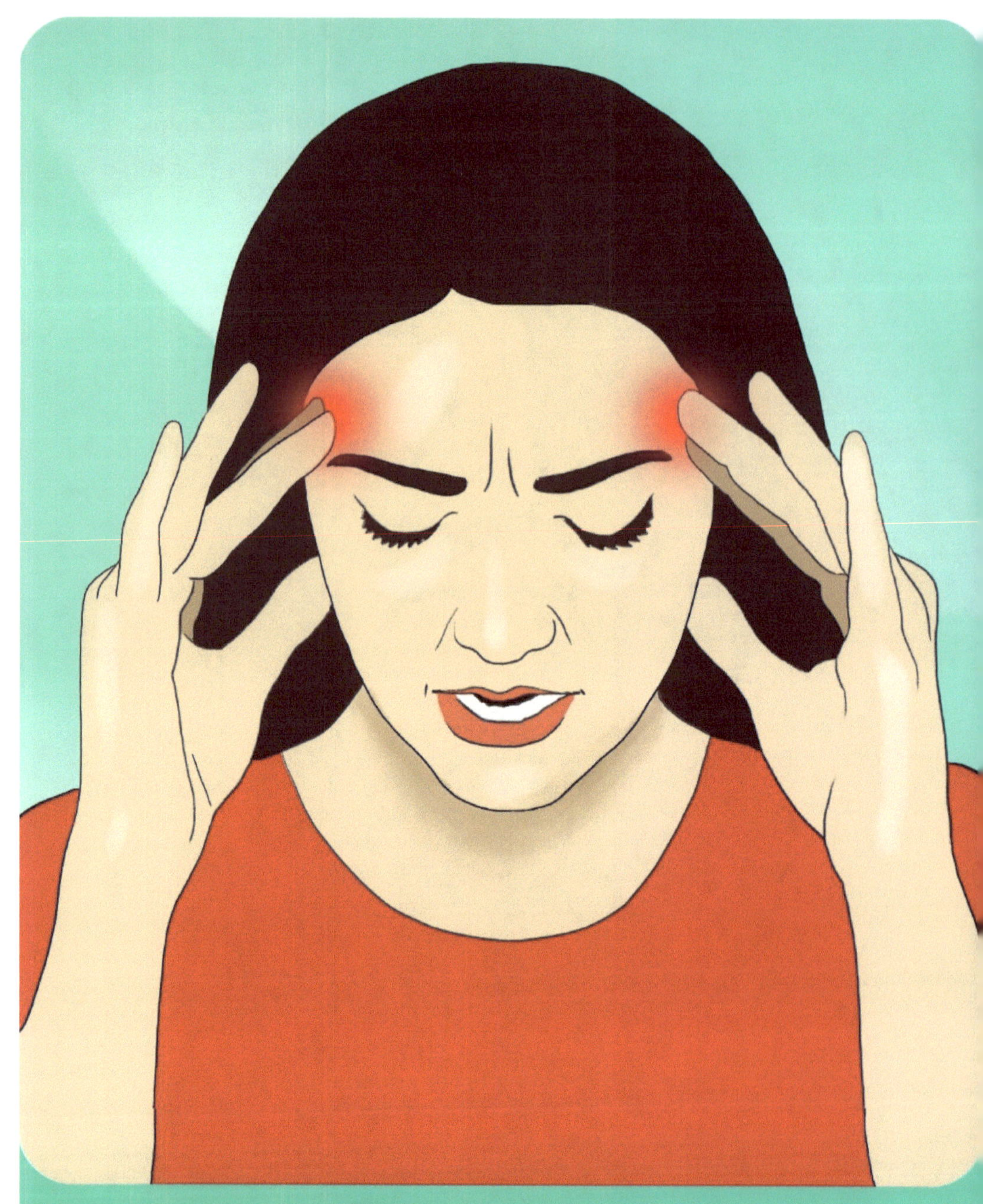

Fewer
migraine attacks

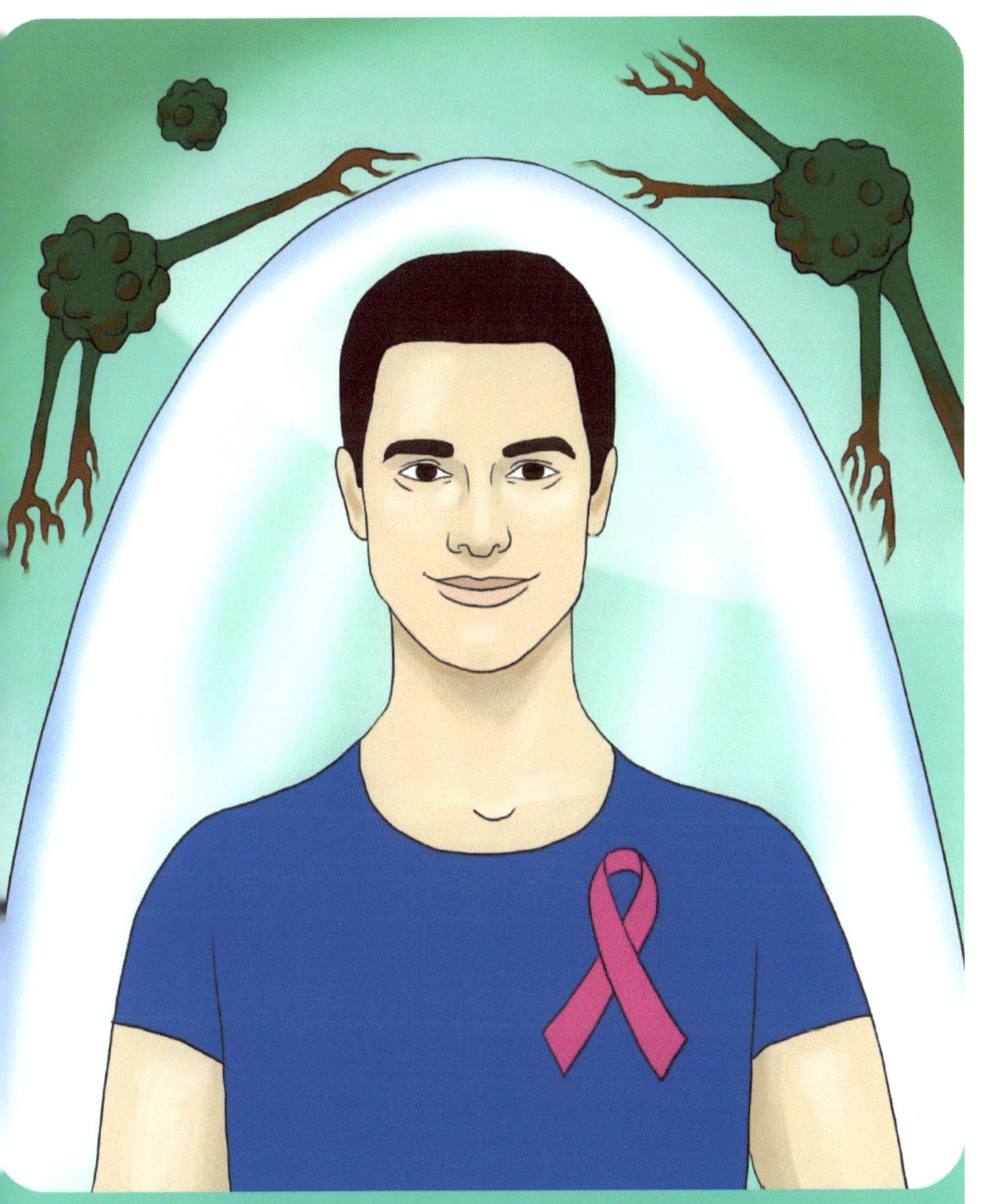

Weakens
cancer cells

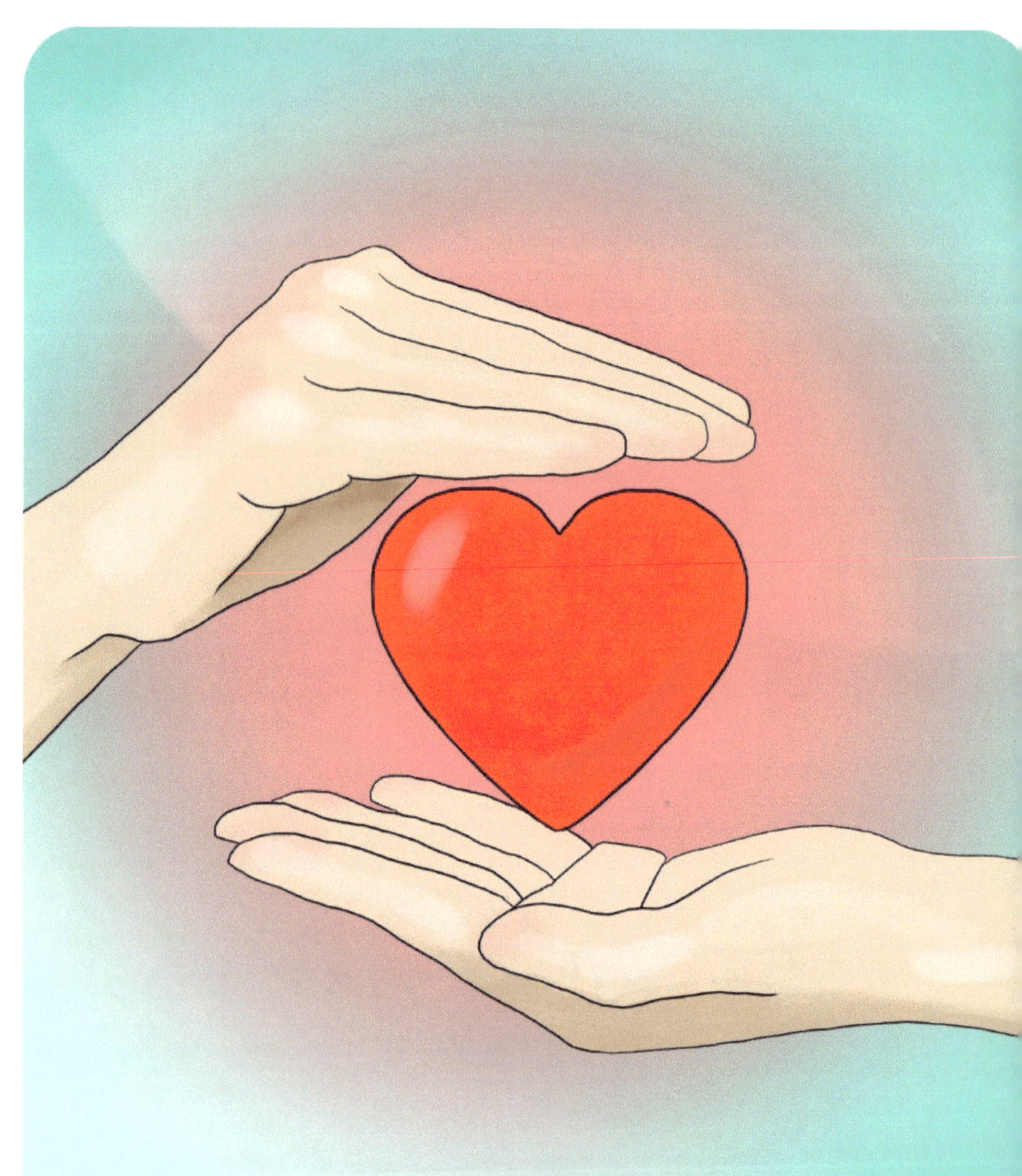

Improve your
heart health

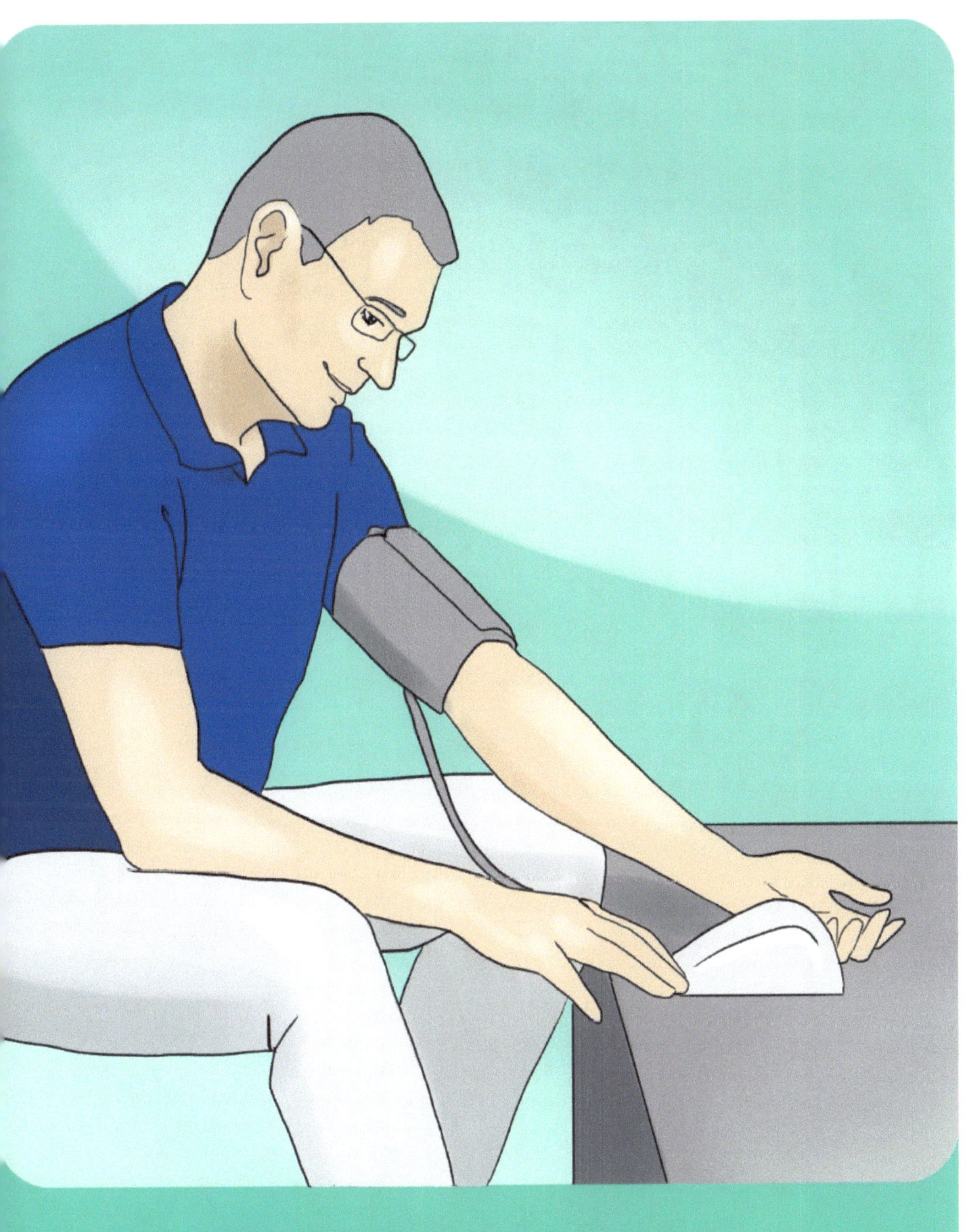

Normalize blood pressure

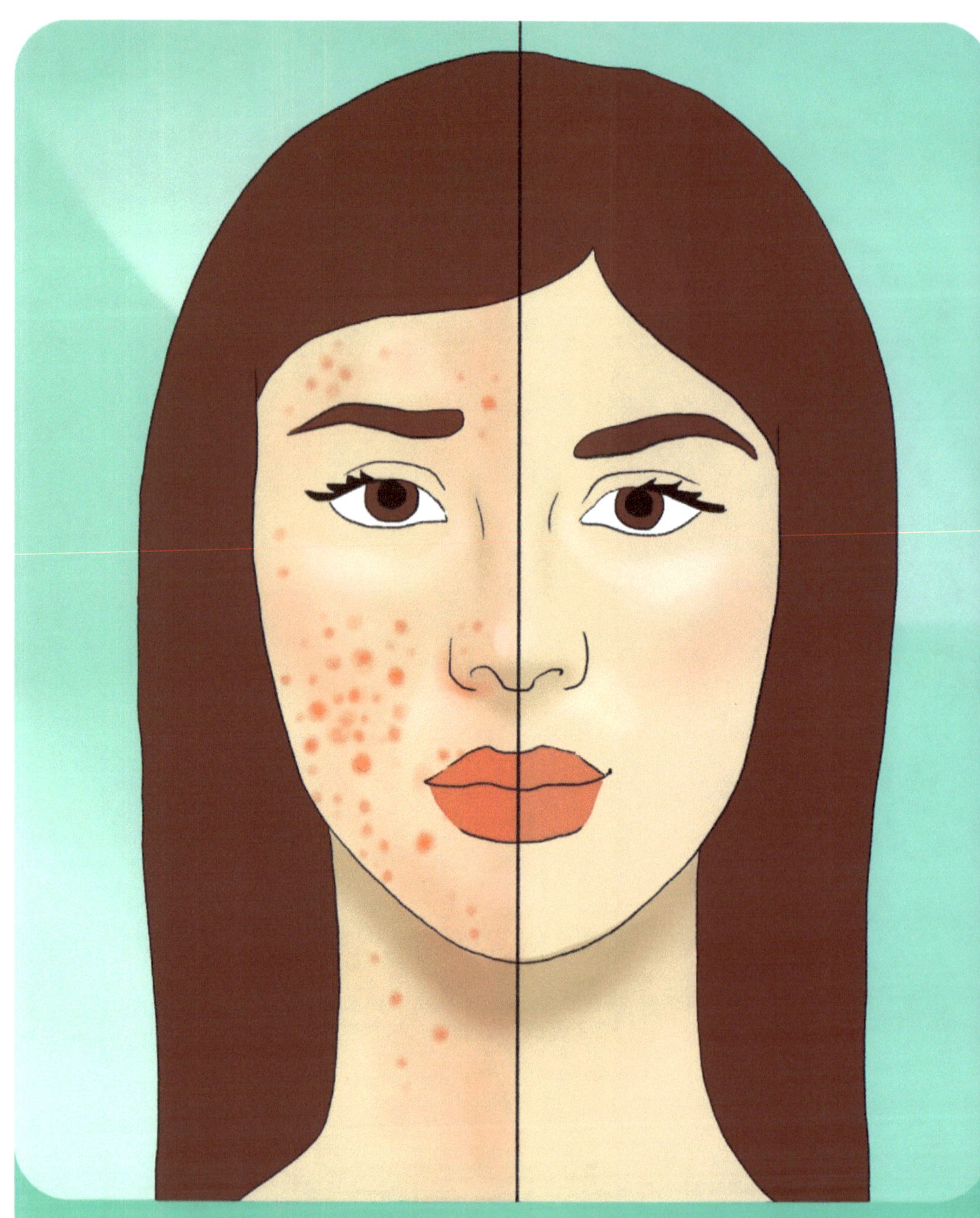

Less acne

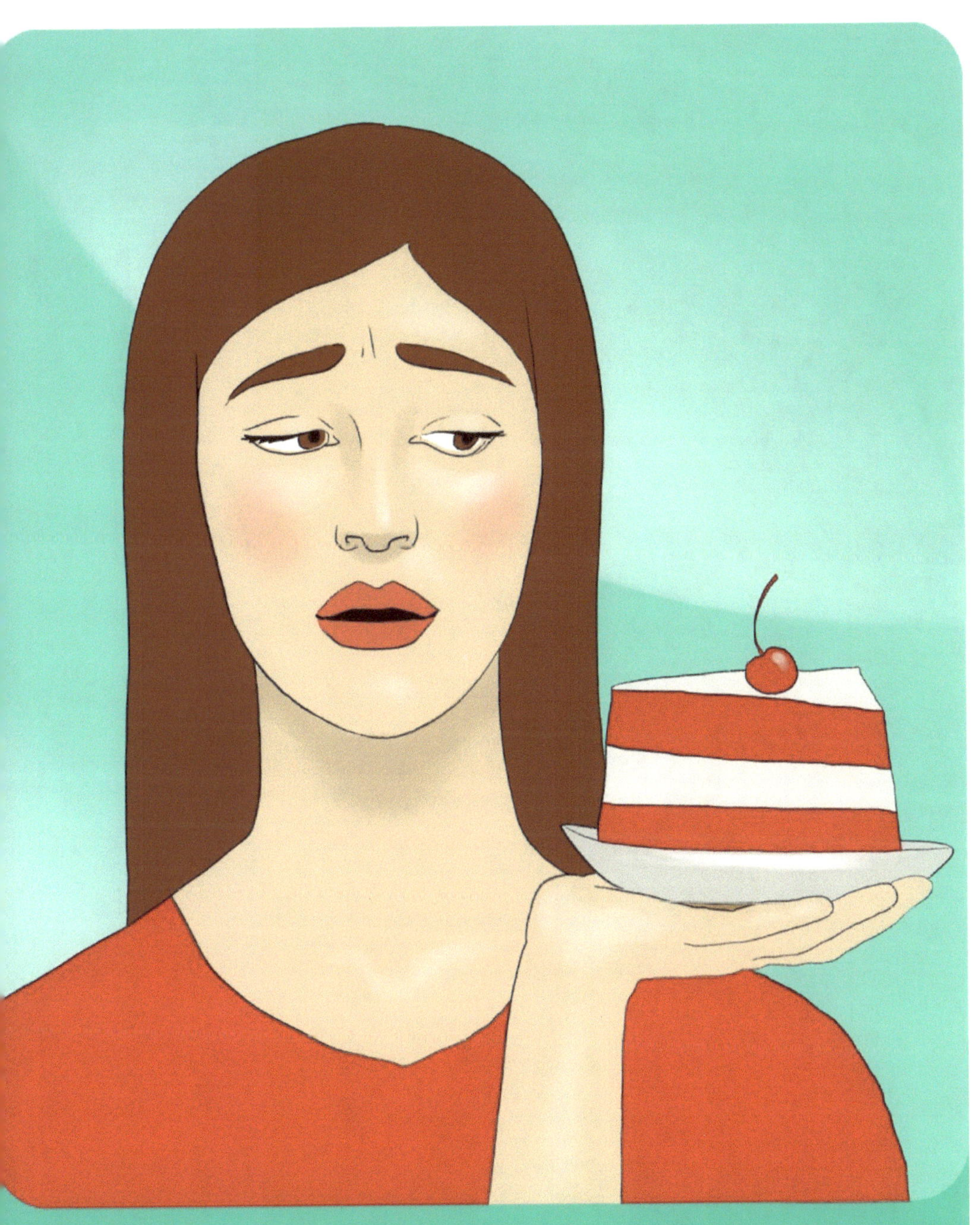

Less
sugar cravings

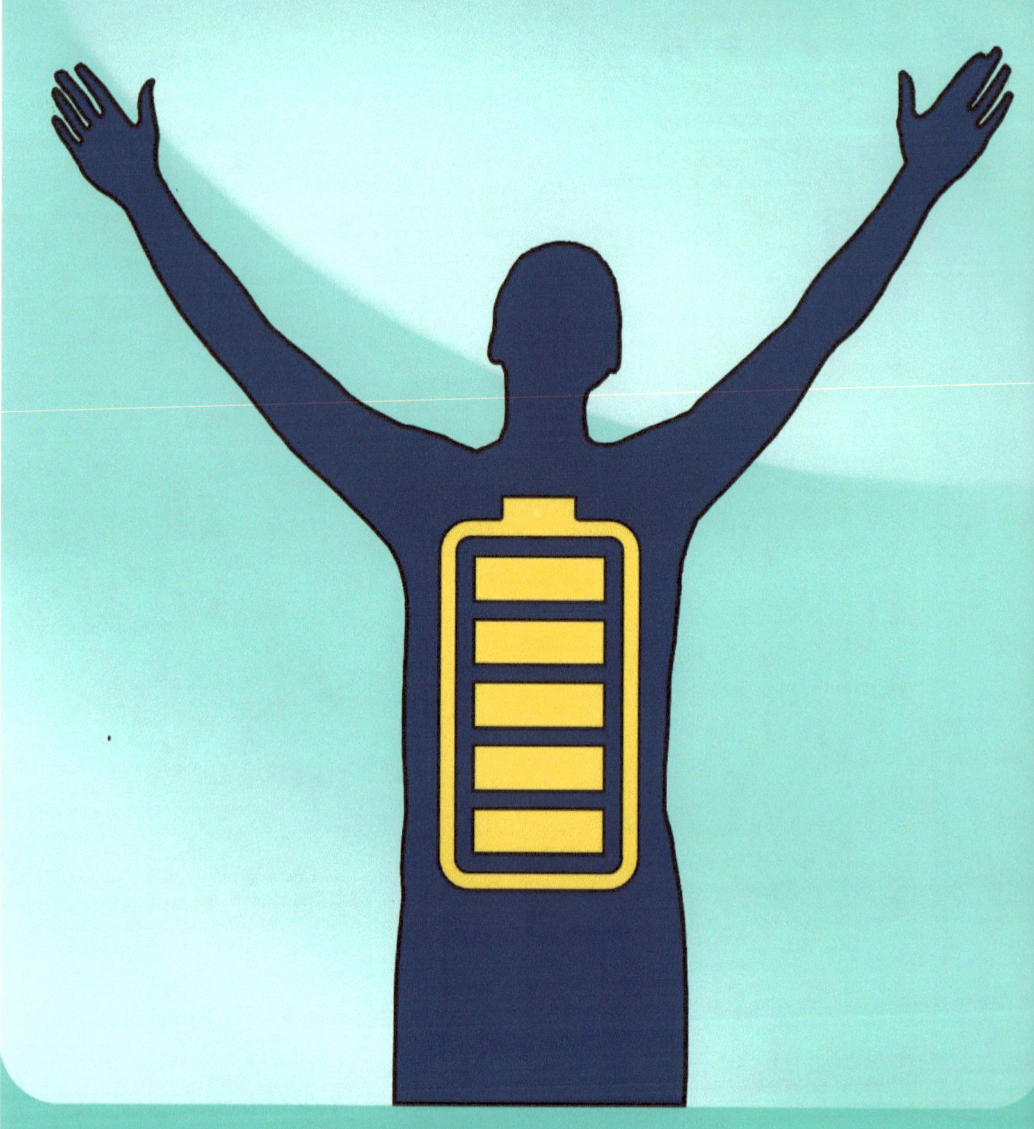

Restore
your energy

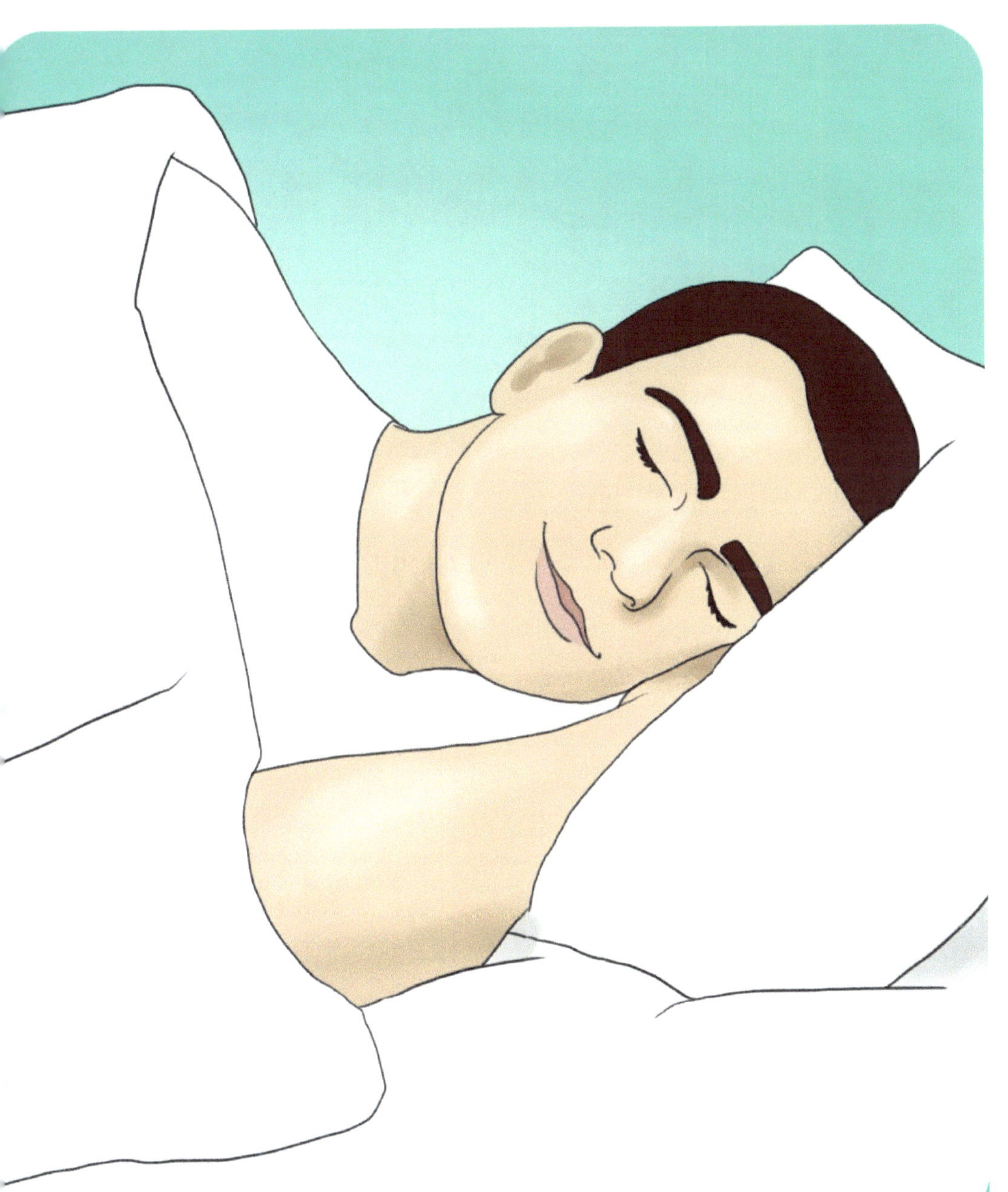

Restful sleep

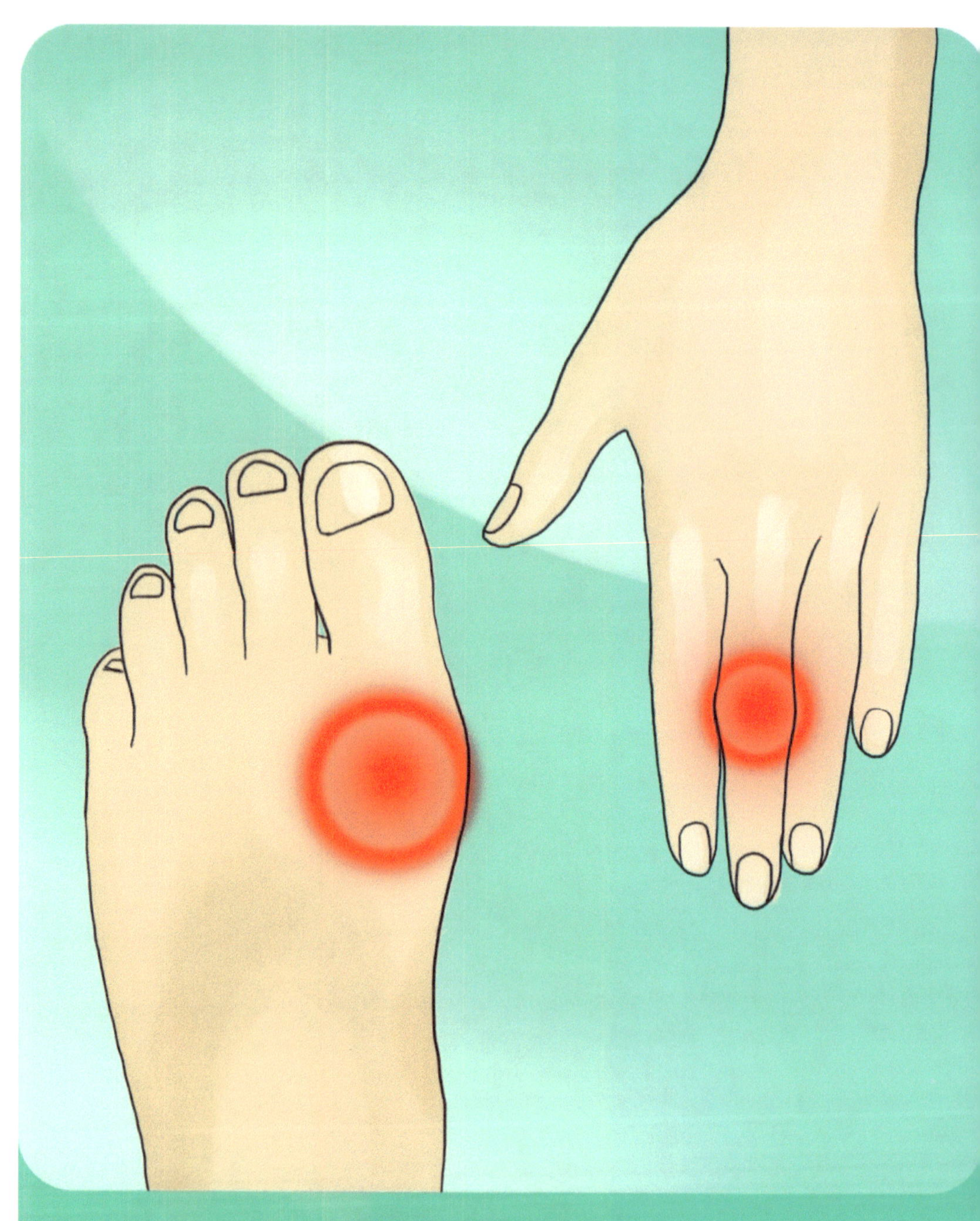

Helps
prevent a gout

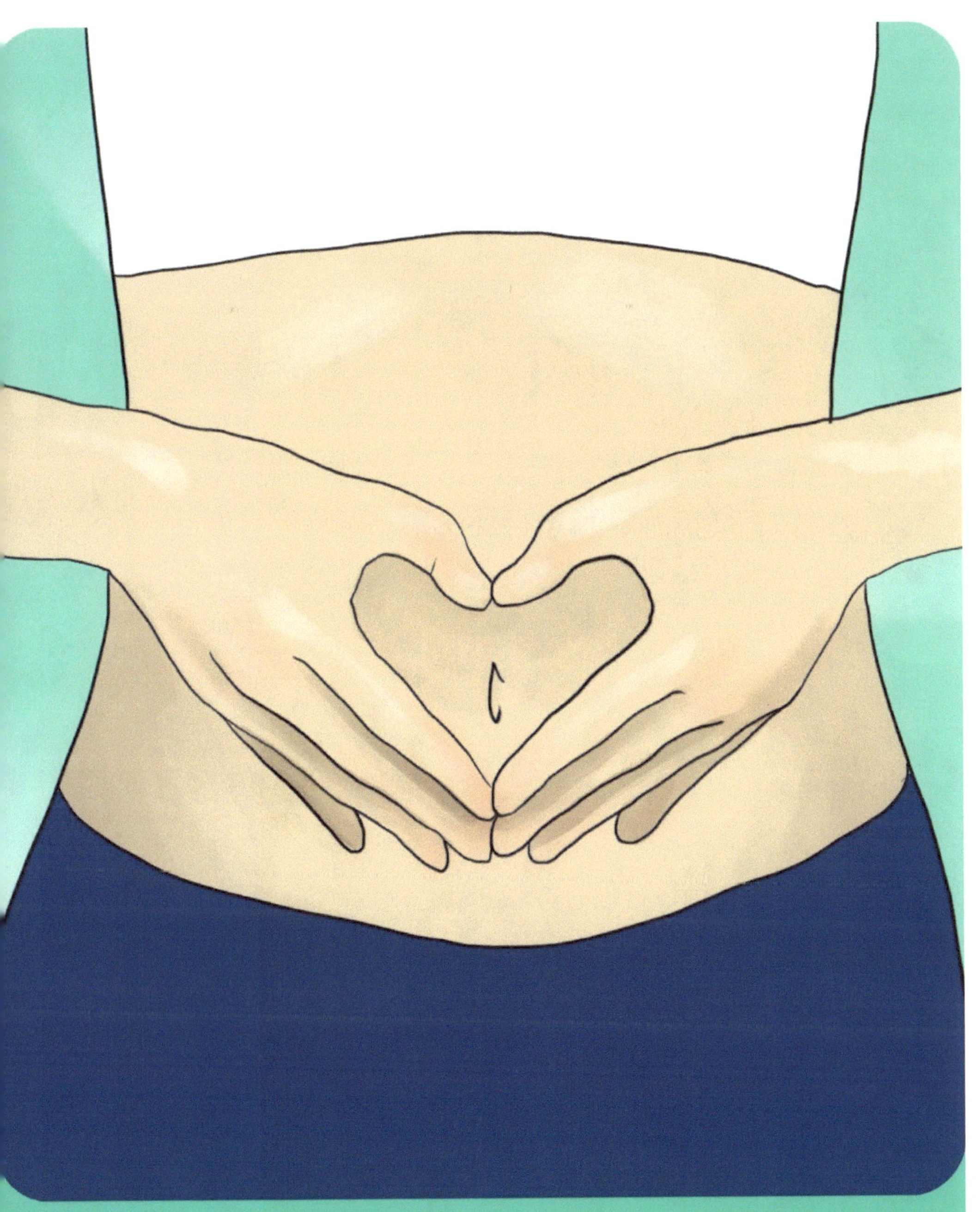

Calm stomach

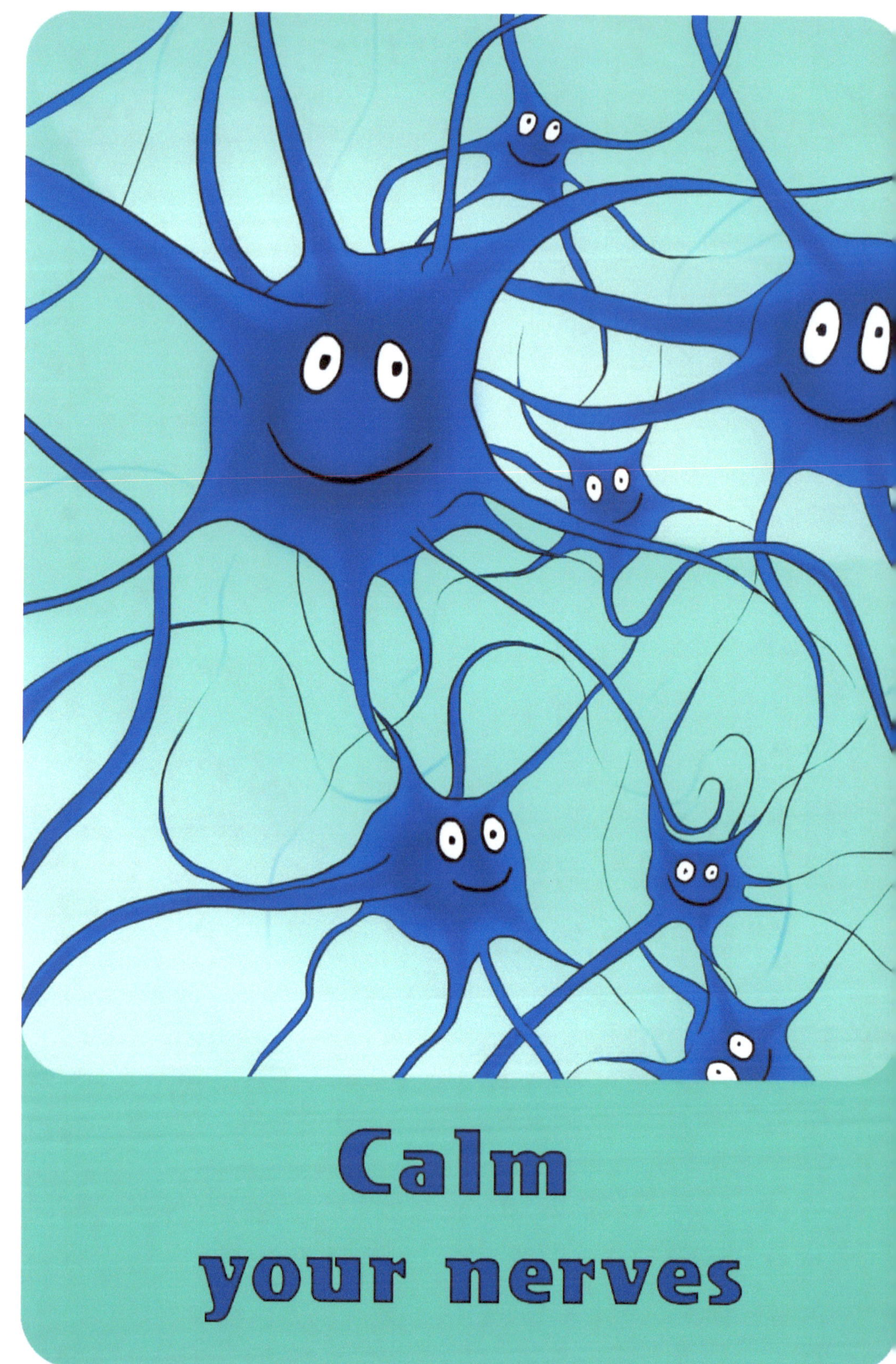
Calm
your nerves

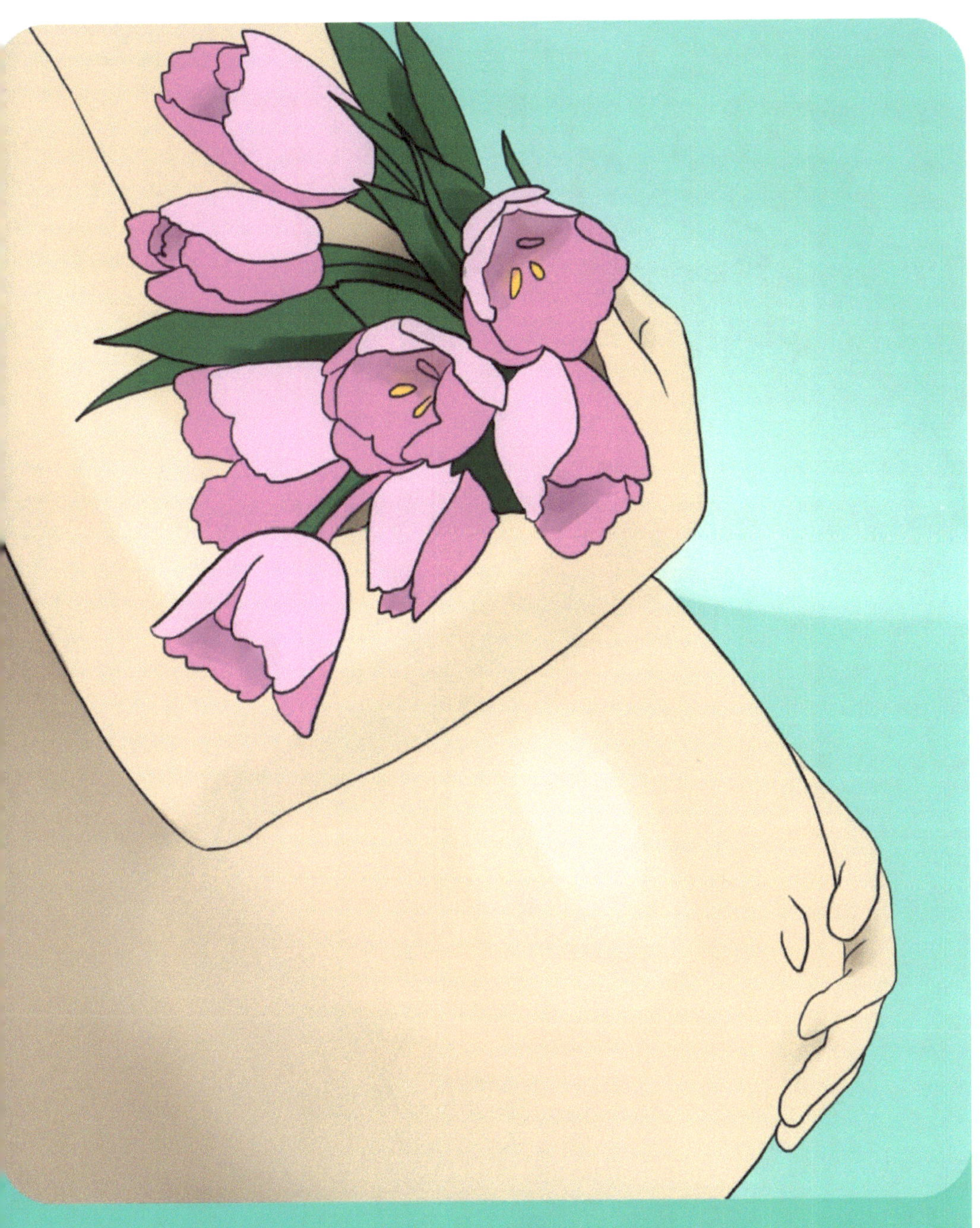

Care about
women's health

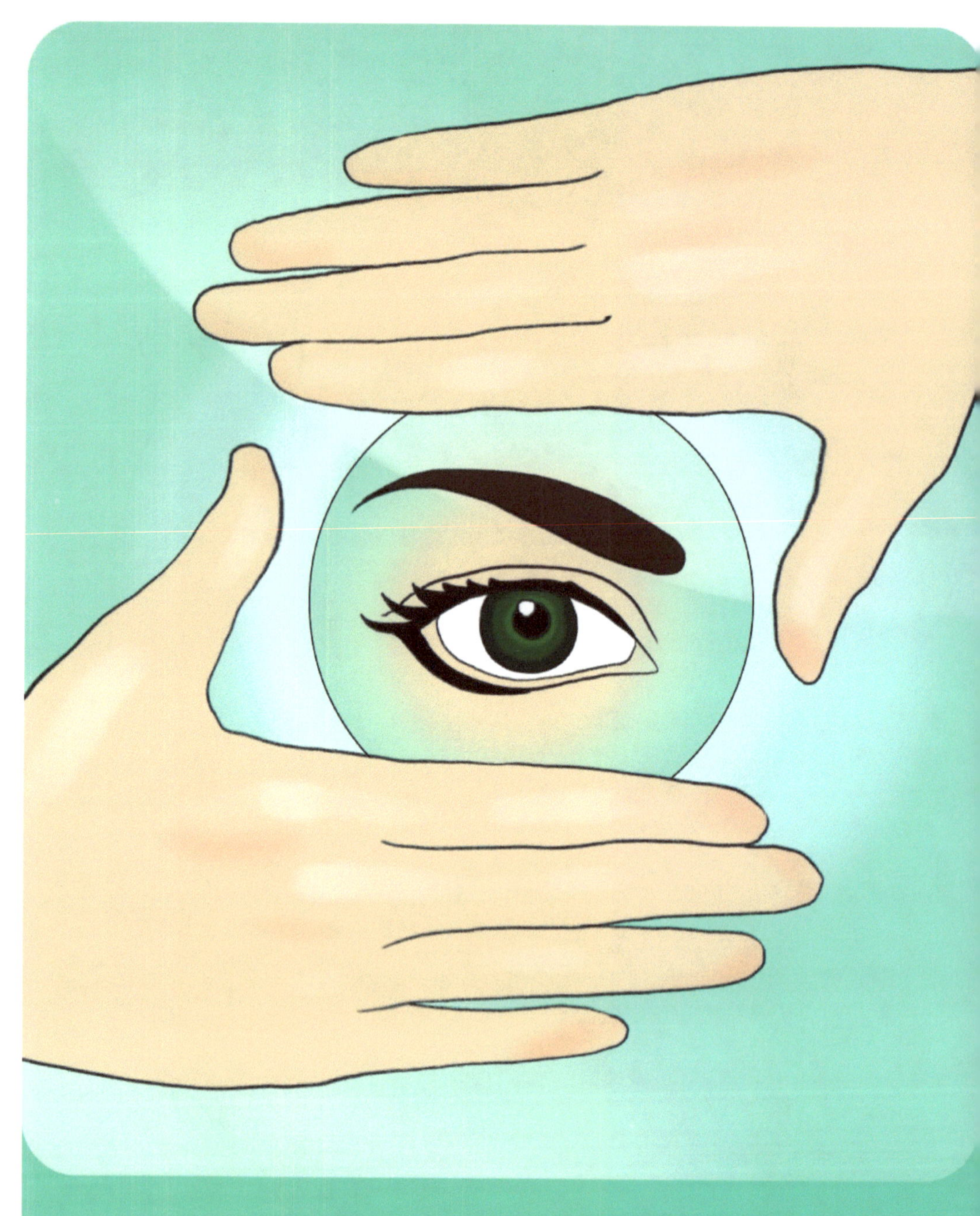

Improve
your eyesight

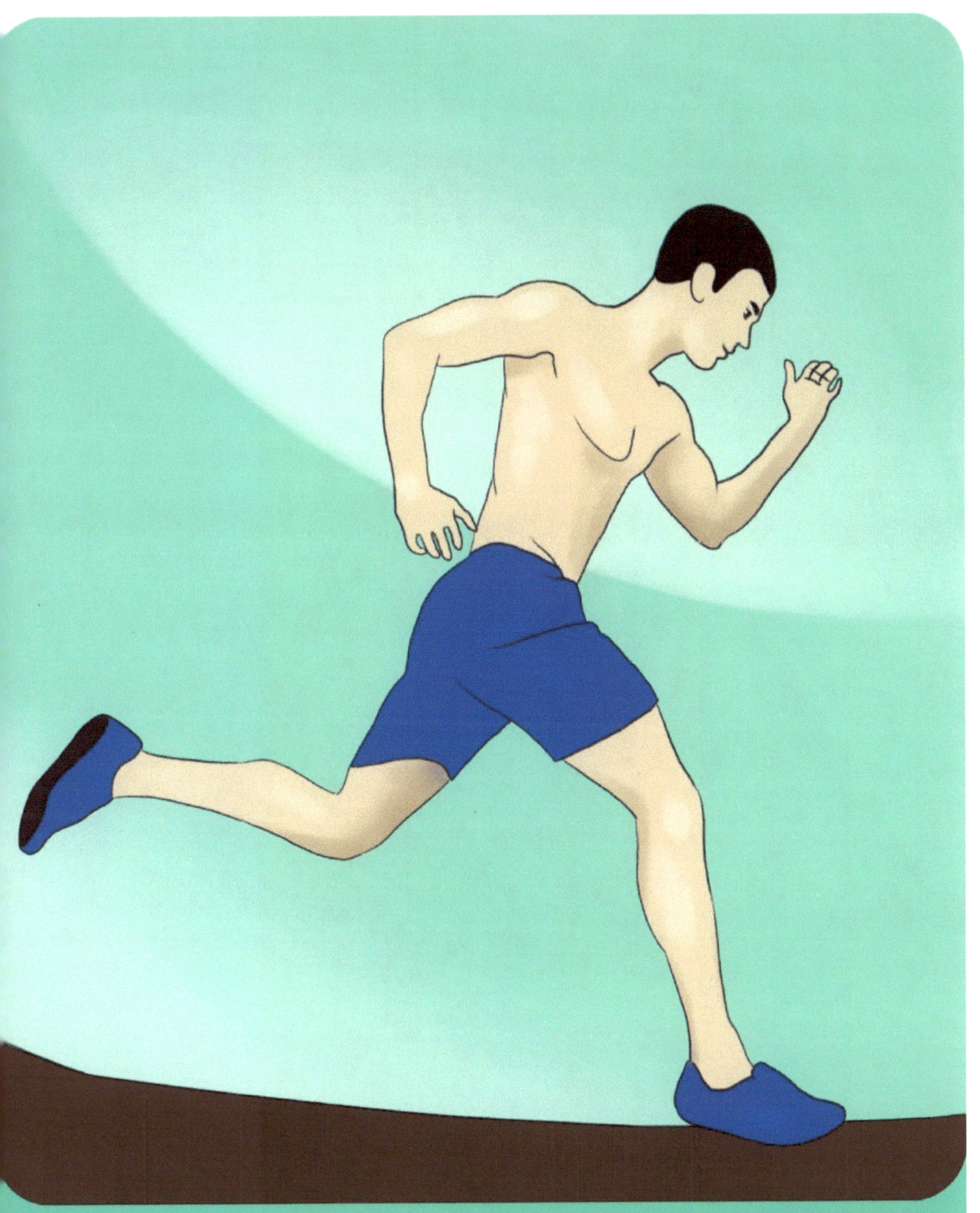

Increased physical
endurance

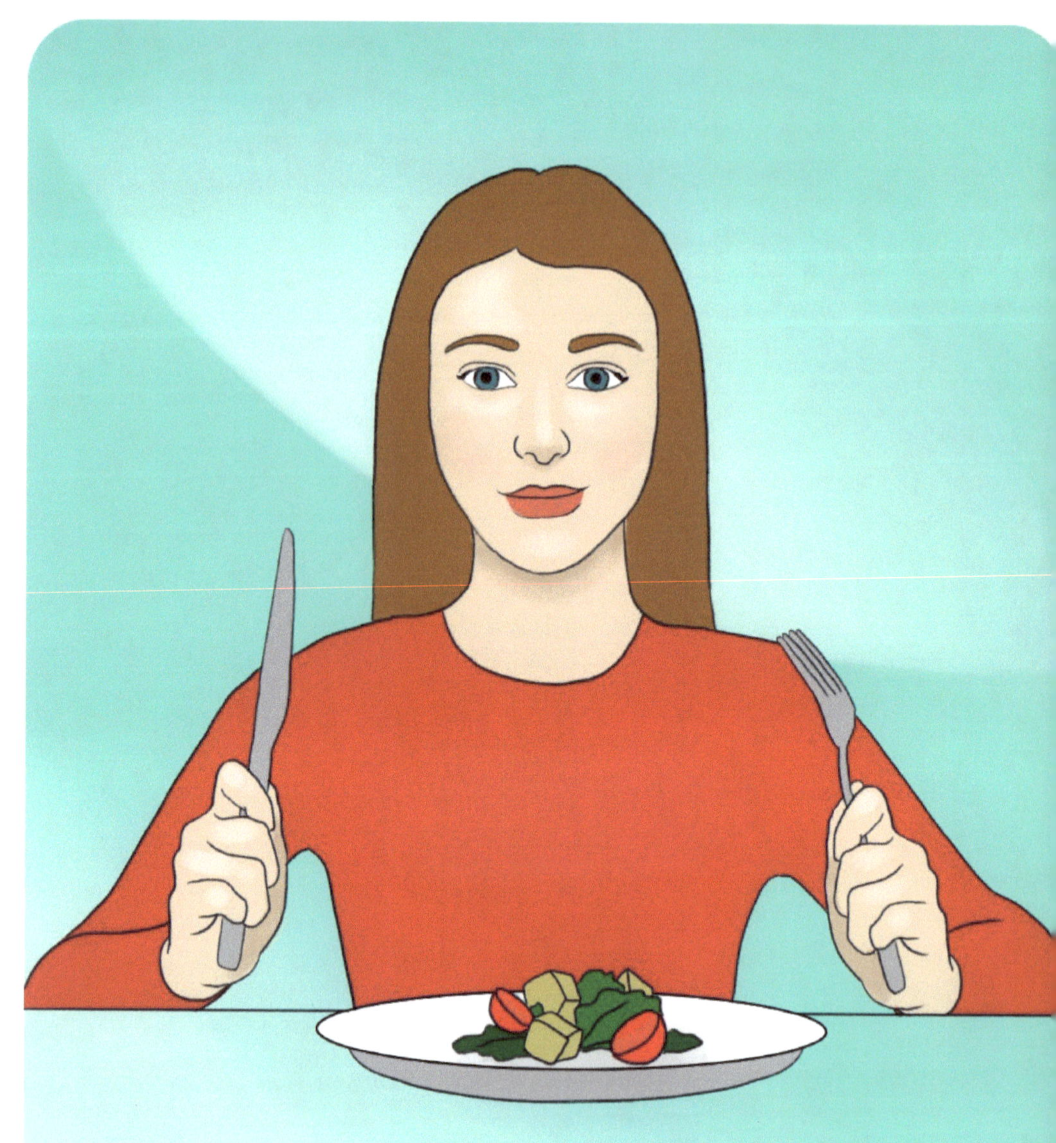

Reduce hunger and lower food intake

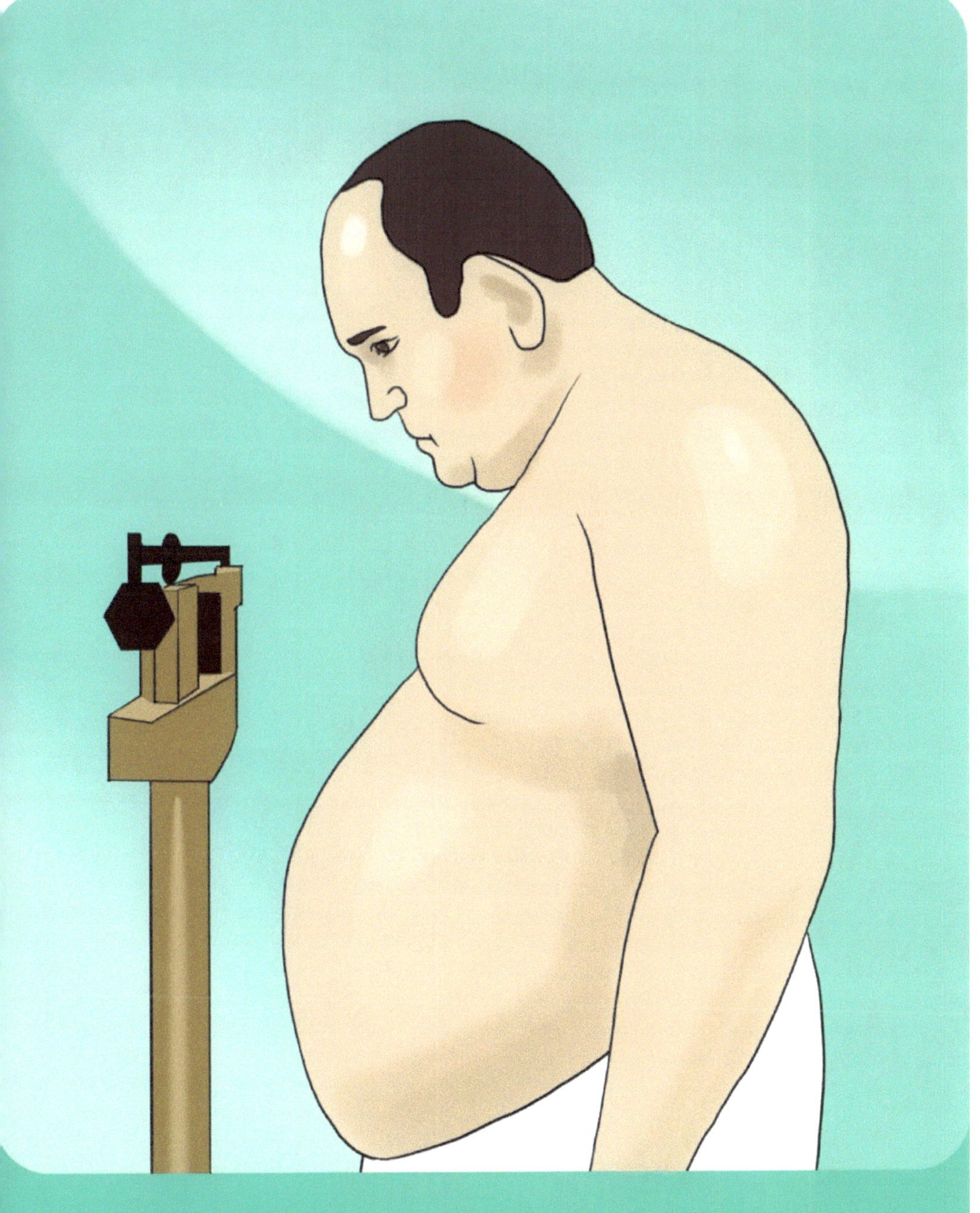

Burn belly fat

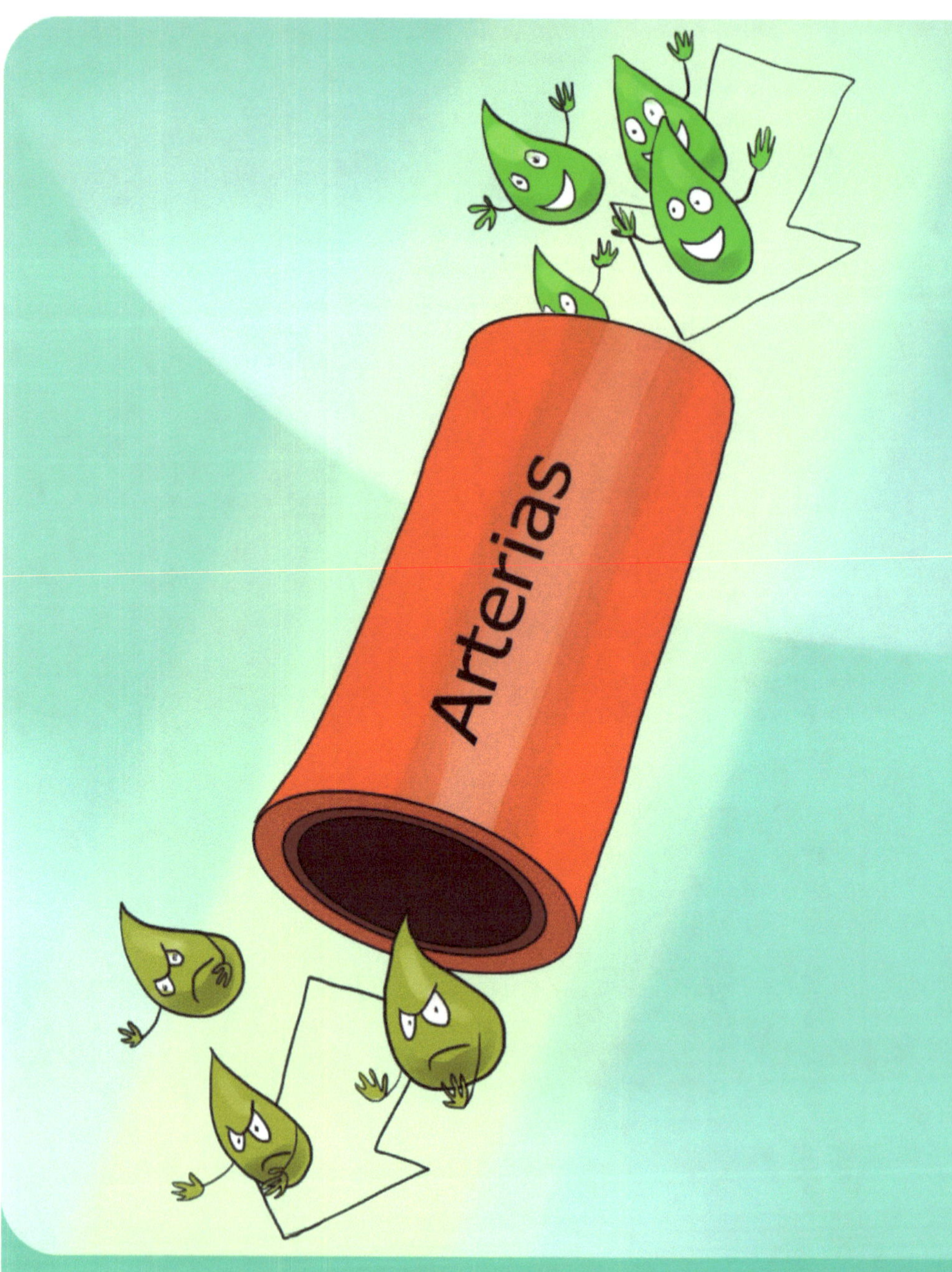

Lower LDL cholesterol

Does it really work?
Yes!

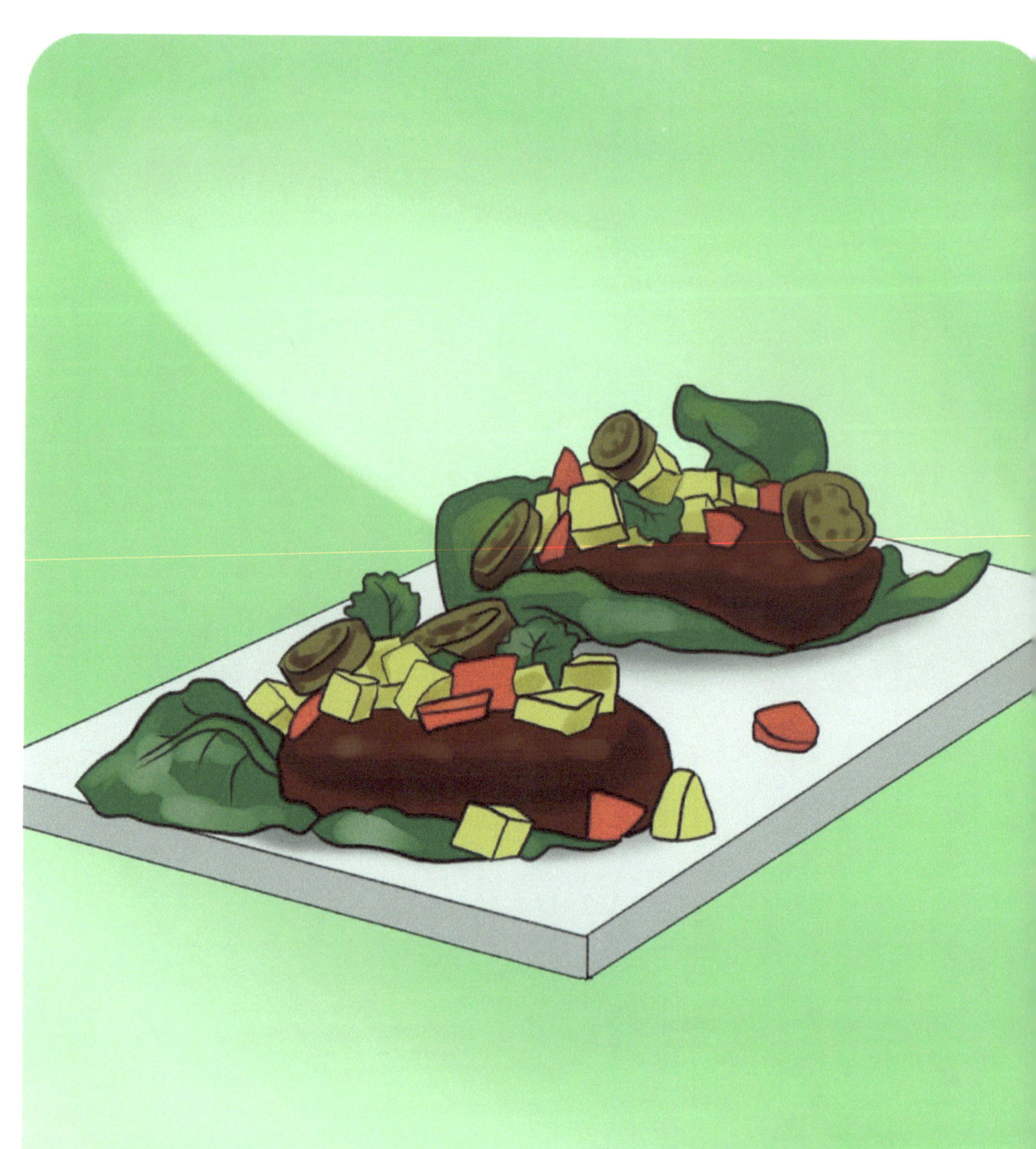

Just eat real food

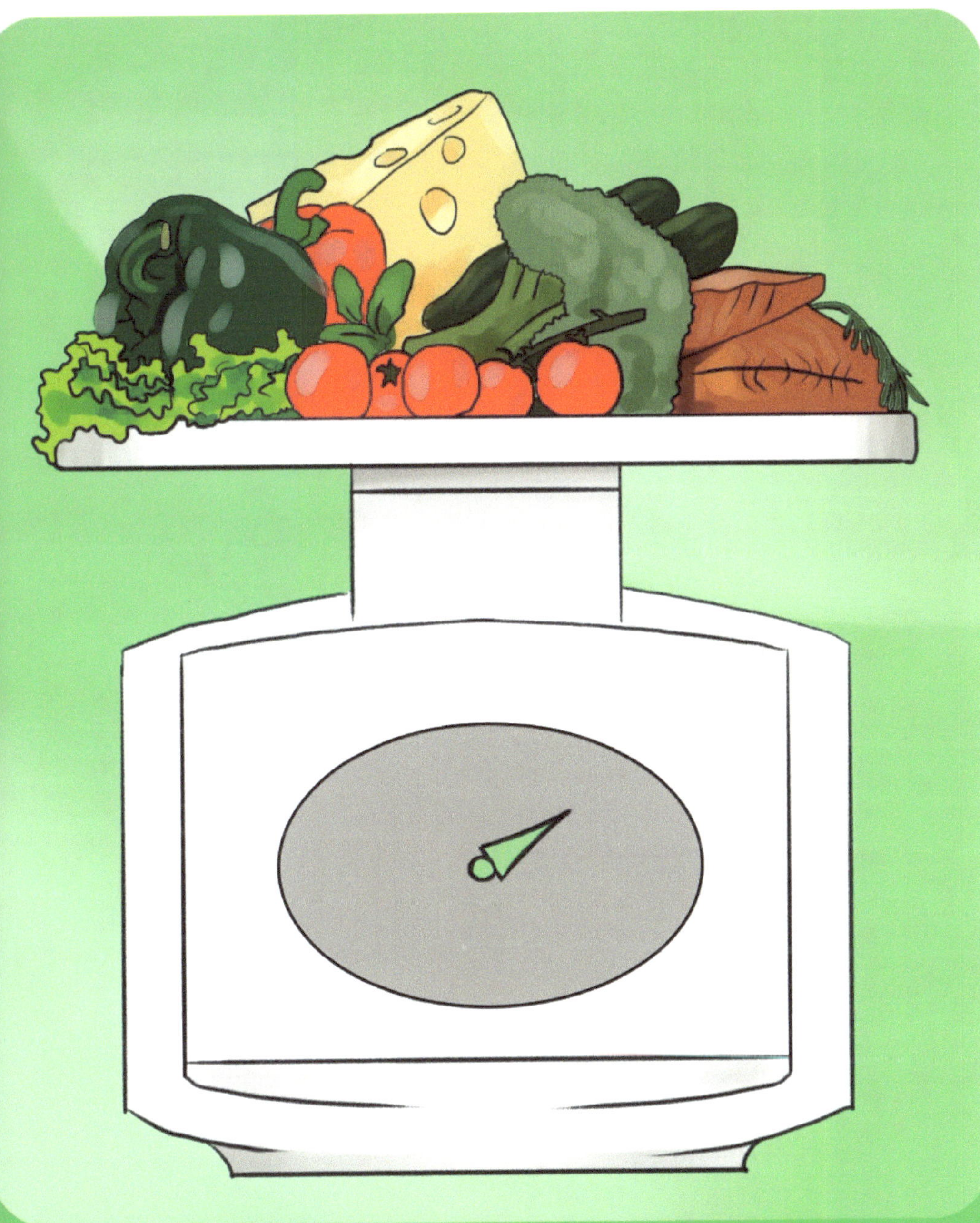

No calorie restrictions

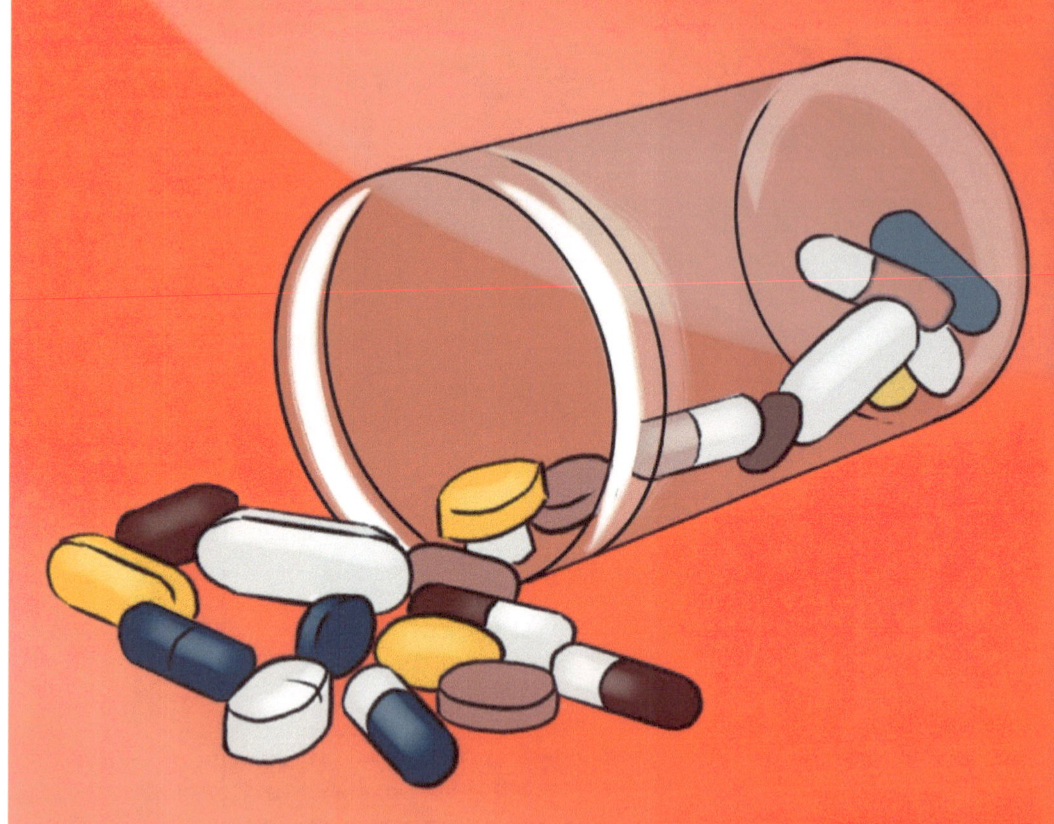

No pills

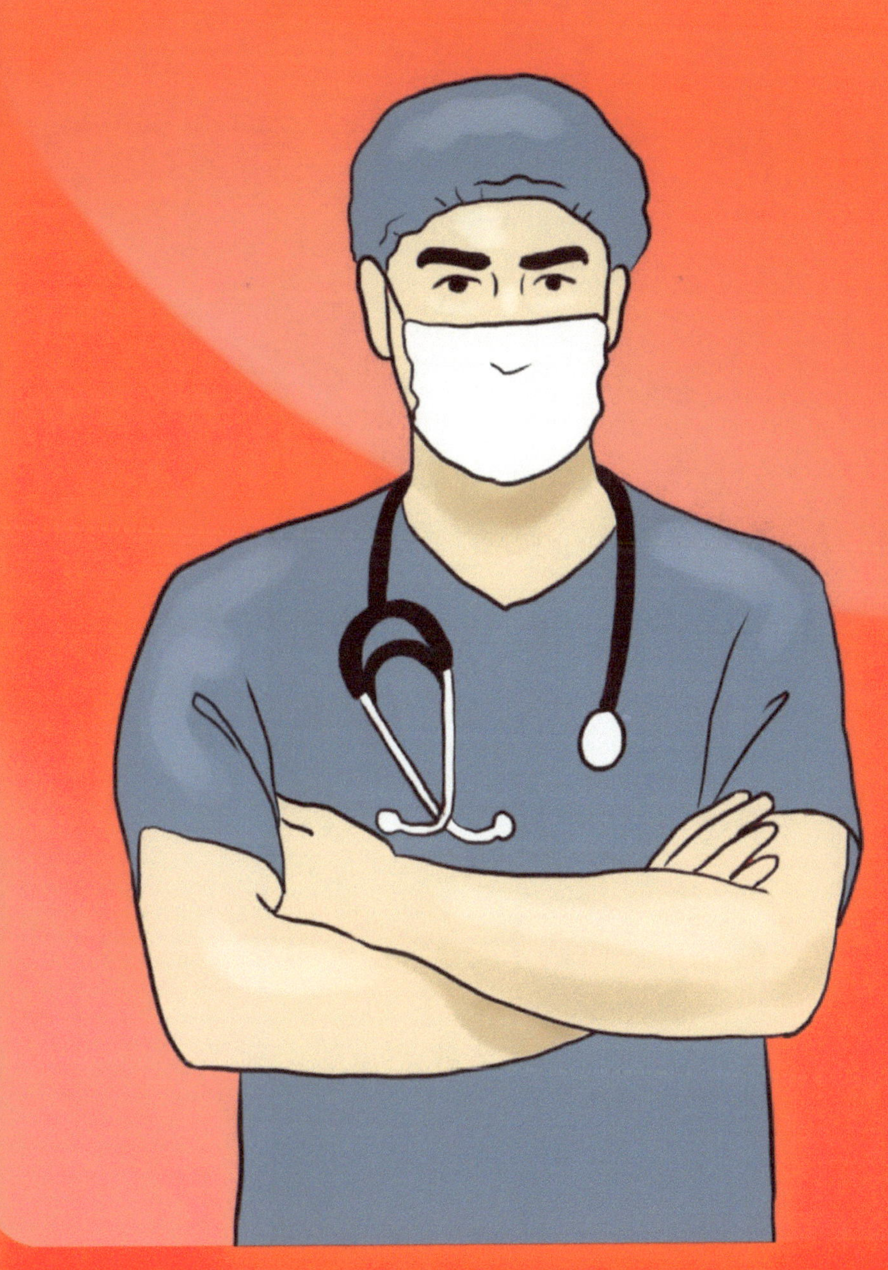

No surgery

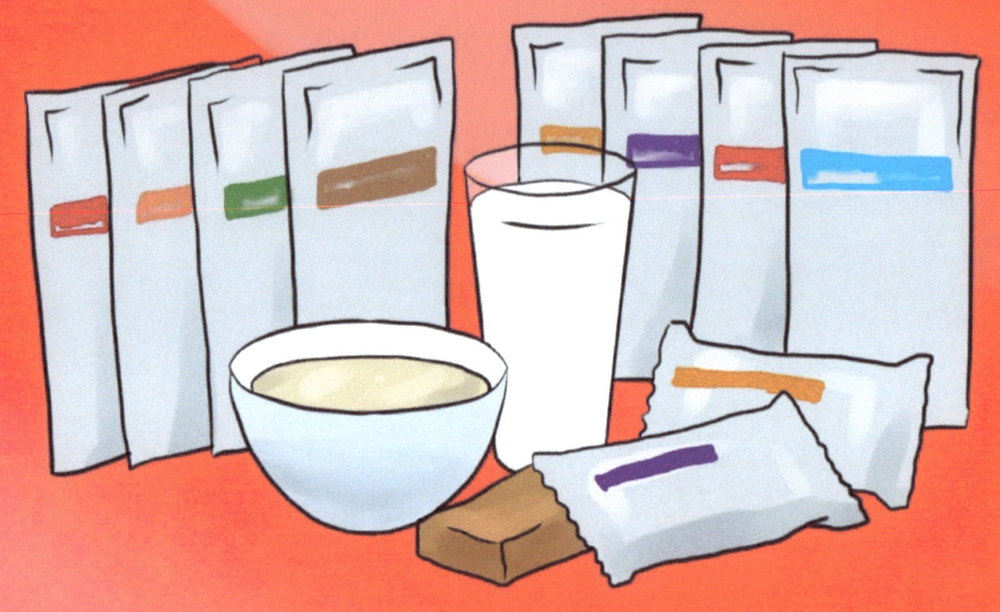

No meal replacements or other fake foods

What processes occur in me?

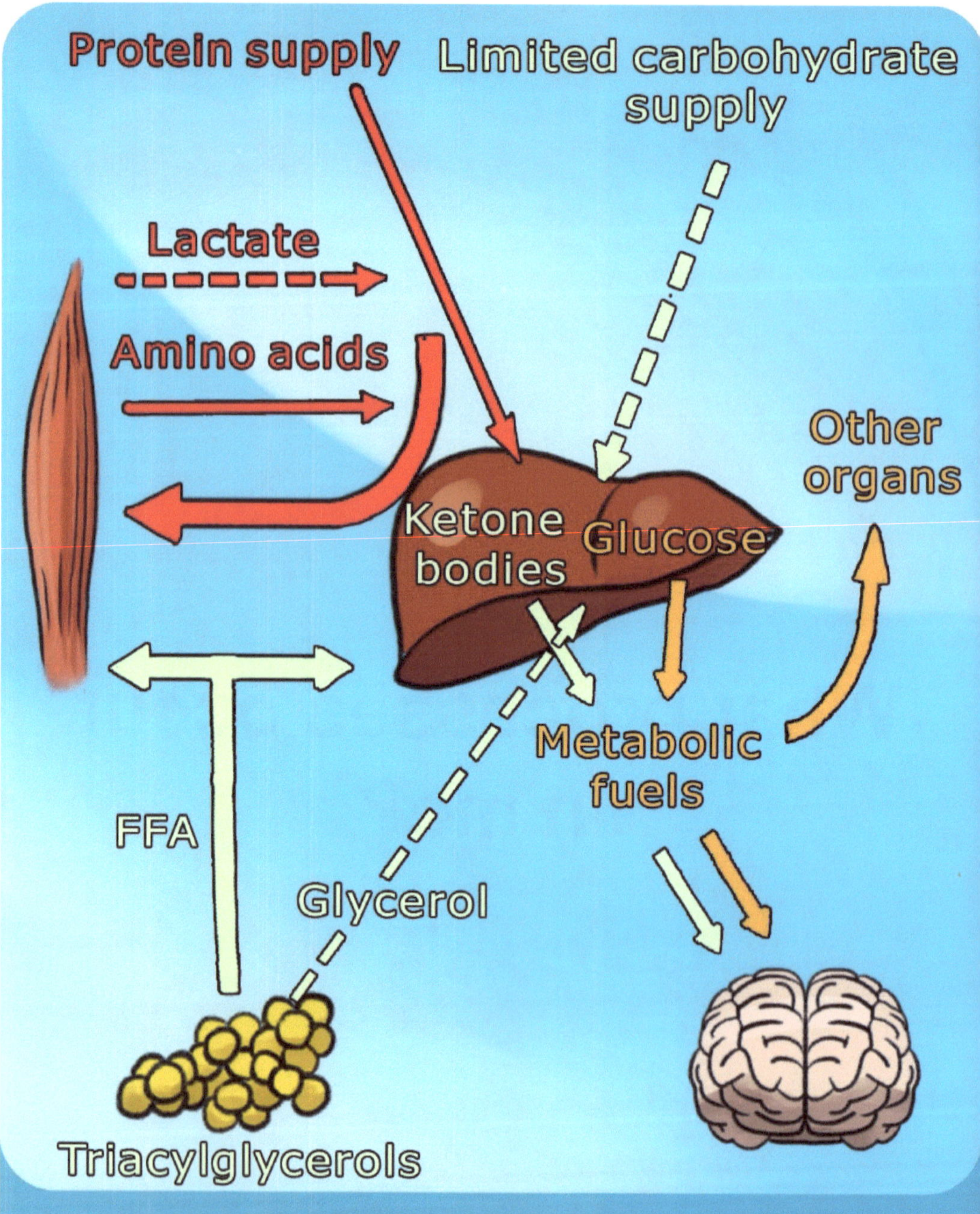

Protein supply
Limited carbohydrate supply
Lactate
Amino acids
Other organs
Ketone bodies
Glucose
Metabolic fuels
FFA
Glycerol
Triacylglycerols
How It All Works?

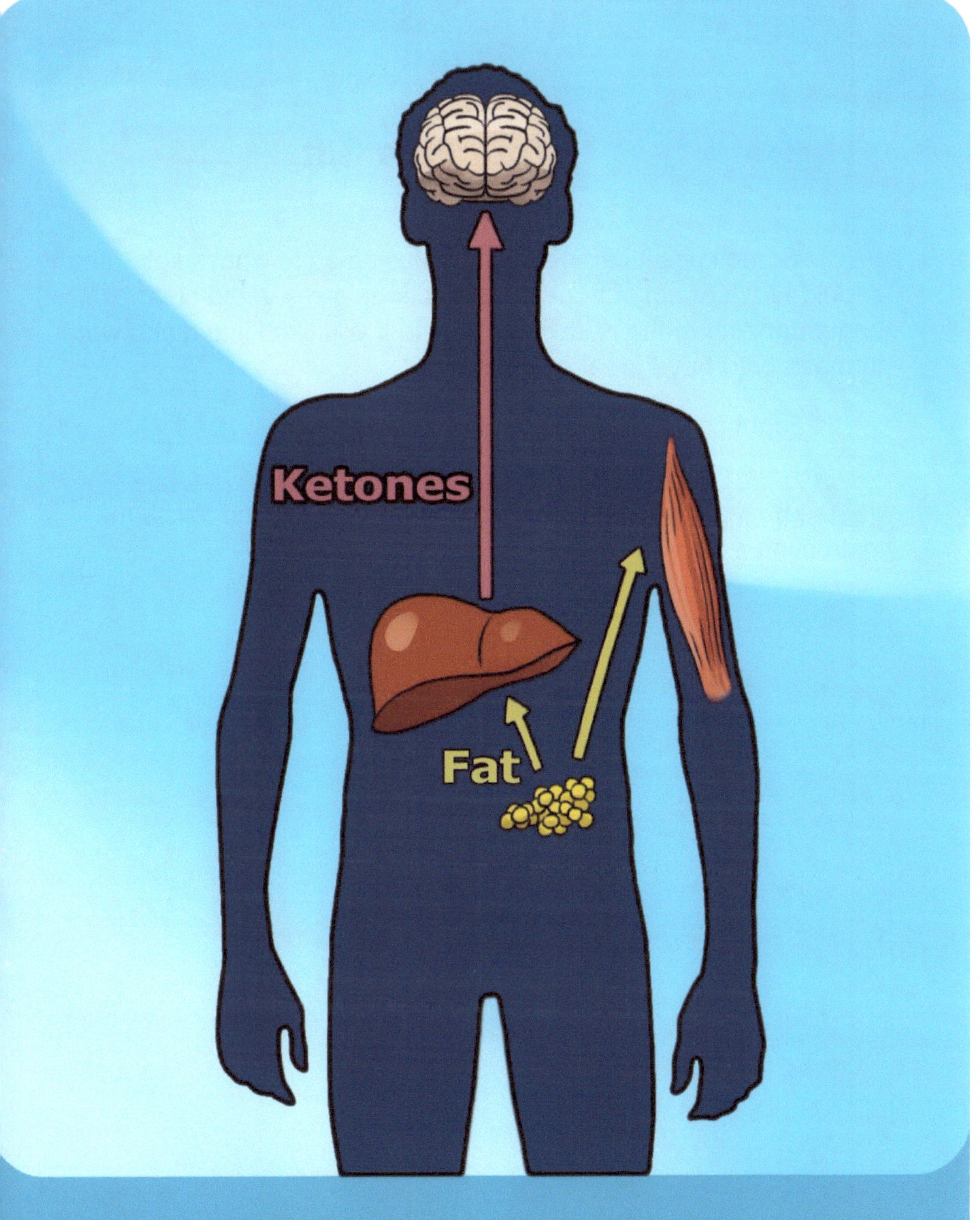

How to achieve ketosis?

Your Free Gift

Sometimes it can get a bit confusing as to what's keto, and should I try it or not? I hope my short book gives you a clear understanding of the Keto's world. And if you liked it and you want to move on, I have great news for you!

Right now, I'm writing a full **Ketogenic Diet For Beginners' guide** and **cookbook**, and if you want to get the books right away, please click on this link and follow the instructions.

Thanks!

Alena Bri